T0149857

The
Nontoxic Baby

**REDUCING HARMFUL CHEMICALS
FROM
YOUR BABY'S LIFE**

NATURAL CHOICES
PUBLISHERS
VISTA, CA 92085
USA

Distributed by
LOTUS LIGHT PUBLICATIONS
Box 325, Twin Lakes, WI 53181
414/889-8561

Text printed on recycled stock with soybean ink

To Concerned Parents

Dear Parents,

You may have not considered that your child simply does not live in the same world as when you or I were born. Approximately **70,000 new chemicals** worldwide have been introduced since WW II, while a thousand new chemicals are still being added each year. Likewise, in 1950, the U.S. production of chemicals was about 1 billion pounds a year. By the 1980's it was over **400 billion pounds** each year. Moreover, approximately 80% of the 48,000 chemicals currently registered with the EPA have virtually no studies on toxic human effects. Undeniably, from the first few seconds of life, our children are the first to truly live in such a chemical world.

I have no trouble believing that these common, daily chemicals can greatly impair health. Just three years, ago, I became critically ill as the result of the toxic chemicals outgassing from my new home and from my bi-monthly pest control service. **All of my chemical exposures were no more than what is commonly referred to as "too minute to cause any harm".** After being completely incapacitated for nearly a year, I am now a person with multiple chemical sensitivities. That means I have mild to life-threatening adverse reactions to many everyday chemicals. According to the National Academy of Sciences, approximately 15-20% of the population has some level of chemical sensitivity—although the connection between chemical exposures and symptoms may not even be known to many of those affected.

Today, the health effect of daily chemicals in our lives is often debated. Some experts actually question the seriousness of this problem, while other experts emphatically state that these toxic chemicals trigger chronic health conditions, changes in behavior, cancer, birth defects and more. As the debate continues, today's parents are faced with many important decisions. Yet as parents, we are not obligated to wait for unaminous perspective in order to provide our children with the healthiest, safest environment possible. Nor do we have to give up our present lifestyle, since we can easily substitute nontoxic products for toxic products. Moreover, when we choose safe products for our families, we also help ensure the future of this planet. Not surprisingly, products which are healthy for humans are also healthy for the earth.

With these thoughts in mind, I enthusiastically welcome you to the world of natural living. I promise, your baby will love you for it!

Nancy Sokol Green

Author of *Poisoning Our Children: Surviving in a Toxic World*. May 1991, The Noble Press, Inc.

Table of Contents

Foreword to Concerned Parents

CHAPER 4

Your Baby's Food .... 4 - 1

CHAPTER 5

Medicine and Your Child .... 5 - 1

Chemical Glossary

Ten chemicals to which we are commonly exposed

Bibliography

Words for parents of the 90's

Active ingredient

The ingredient in a pesticide formula intended to kill the targeted pest.

Acute effects

Symptoms that happen almost immediately after exposure.

Chronic effects

Symptoms that result after repeated exposures, developing over a period of time.

Detoxification system

The body's internal system which removes toxins.

EPA

Environmental Protection Agency.

FDA

Food and Drug Administration.

Inert Ingredient

Ingredients used as solvents, emulsifiers, conditioning agents, etc. in pesticide formulations.

Masking

The body's ability to initally cover up symptoms - even though the body is still being stressed.

OSHA

Occupational Safety and Health Administration.

Outgassing

An on-going, invisible evaporation from solid materials. When products are new, chemical vapors are often smelled (e.g. new carpet). However, the outgassing process continues long past our olfactory ability to detect it.

Sensitivities

An adverse reaction to a food or chemical even when exposed to very small amounts.

Synergistic Effect

When chemicals combine together to produce an effect which is different and greater than either chemical alone.

Toxin

The Greek word for poison.

How chemicals enter your baby's body

Chemicals enter the body by:

Inhalation

Invisible chemical vapors are inhaled through the mouth and nose; these vapors may or may not be smelled.

Ingestion

Chemicals enter the body through the digestive tract.

Skin absorption

Chemicals enter the body through contact with the skin, a porous permeable membrane.

Why be concerned

Recurrent Ear Infections

Today, recurrent ear infections result in approximately one million children a year having surgery to place tubes inside their ears.

Asthma

In 1985, one of every five children with asthma was hospitalized.

Asthma is now the leading cause of pediatric hospitalizations.

Between 1983 and 1987, asthma death rates rose by 30% in the United States.

In 1989, 12 million people had asthma compared to 6 million in 1970.

Hyperactive Children

Approximately 30% of school children are now labeled as hyperactive.

The use of Ritalin and other related drugs to treat hyperactivity has doubled every 4-7 years.

Medicated hyperactive boys are considered to be a high risk for problems at school and with the law.

75% of all prisoners today were hyperactive children.

Formaldehyde

Nine billion pounds of formaldehyde are produced annually.

Formaldehyde is basic to 77 industries and accounts for approximately 8% of the gross national product.

Formaldehyde is in over 85 common household items.

A preliminary study has indicated that formaldehyde may play a contributory role in *Sudden Infant Death Syndrome.*

Formaldehyde causes cancer in test animals.

In 1987, the EPA announced that formaldehyde probably also causes cancer in humans.

Daily exposure to formaldehyde can cause many symptoms such as: *watery eyes, bronchitis, chronic ear infections, and asthma..*

Food

Over one half of all the food on grocery store shelves has only appeared within the last decade.

In another 10 years, that number is predicted to be as high as 80%.

60% of the population is now believed to have some food sensitivities.

Food companies can create committees which are many times cited as sources of food safety.

> *Examples:*
>
> *The National Academy of Science Food Protection Committee*

(independently financed by commercial labs, packaging and chemical companies)

The Nutrition Foundation, Inc. (whose directors are not limited to The American Sugar Company, Coca-cola, Beechnut, Campbell Soup, and General Mills)

Impossible Testing Expectations

Since 1981, most of the existing regulations protecting the public from toxic chemicals were canceled, postponed or weakened.

Budgets of several federal environmental and consumer protection regulatory agencies were cut by millions in the early 1980's.

In May of 1981, the Consumer Product Safety Commission (CPSC) was also recommended to be completely eliminated.

While the CPSC was not eliminated, this agency suffered severe budget cutbacks.

The CPSC now cannot even begin to test or monitor the countless products appearing on the market today.

Therefore, government has had to rely on manufacturers to do their own testing.

This becomes a legitimate concern to consumers for numerous reasons:

- *400 billion pounds of chemicals are produced each year.*
- *1,000 new chemicals are added each year.*
- *Most testing is usually limited to only acute effects.*
- *The overwhelming majority of products on the market today have rarely (if ever) been tested for chronic or synergistic effects.*

Trade Secrets

Manufacturers are allowed to include trade secret ingredients in product formulations.

In order to protect manufacturers from competitors, these ingredients do not have to be listed on product labels.

These trade secret ingredients can legally comprise as much as 99% of the entire product.

According to EPA reports, many of these trade secret ingredients are toxic chemicals.

Unidentified trade secret ingredients makes it impossible to accurately claim a product's safety.

Indoor Air Contaminants

The EPA did a five year study of indoor air contaminants.

The study showed some homes to have chemical levels seventy times higher than what was detected outdoors.

Not one single government agency monitors the level of indoor pollutants.

Toxic Chemicals in the Body

A study by the EPA found toxic chemicals to be stored in the fat tissues of every person in the study.

100% of the people tested had styrene, xylene, 1-4 Dichlorobenzene, ethylphenol, and dioxin stored in their fat tissue.

55% of the people had DDT stored, even though DDT has been banned since the seventies.

Chemicals and Reproductive Function

In a study done at major universities, 25% of college males were found to be sterile.

This compared to only $1/2$% of college males found to be sterile 35 years ago.

A director of major sperm bank states that in the last 10 years, he has had trouble finding quality sperm donors.

The director claims that he has to turn away 9 out of 10 applicants.

The increase of pesticides, PCBs, and other chemicals in our lives have been indicated as primary reasons for male sterility.

Increased Leukemia Risk

Children exposed to common household pesticides have a 7x greater chance of getting childhood leukemia.

Toxins in the Brain

The brain is a very permeable organ, therefore making it a target organ of many chemicals.

Symptoms which can result from a cerebral reaction to toxins in the brain are (but not limited to) *hyperactivity, moodiness, disorientation,* and *depression.*

Your Baby

Your baby cannot tell you if he or she is reacting to an environmental trigger.

All your baby can do is cry, act irritable, or lethargic.

Even when your child is old enough to verbalize symptoms, he or she may not recognize them as symptoms.

This is because he or she has never had a baseline to know that such reactions are not normal.

Why be encouraged

Nontoxic Alternatives

A wide variety of nontoxic products and alternatives exist for almost every commercial product (associated with toxic chemicals).

Parents

Parents are in the position to easily reduce the number of chemical exposures in their children's lives.

Environmental Medicine

Doctors specializing in environmental medicine are called clinical ecologists.

Clinical ecologists are licensed medical doctors who specialize in *environmental medicine.*

Environmental medicine focuses on the relationship between symptoms and environmental exposures (chemicals, food, molds, etc.).

Environmental medicine offers alternate effective treatment for many previously labeled chronic conditions such as:

Recurrent Ear Infections

Food and chemicals sensitivities are ruled out before ever considering surgery.

For many children, eliminating the offending environmental trigger(s) has ended their chronic recurrent ear infections.

Hyperactive Children

A non-medicated approach has proven to bring remarkable positive behavior changes in many hyperactive children.

Such an approach includes diet changes, reducing chemical exposures, and prescribing nutrient supplements.

Examples:

45 children labeled as hyperactive or as having learning difficulties were studied.

41 out of the 45 demonstrated that their symptoms were triggered by food sensitivities.

28 of the 41 children were sensitive to milk.

With the removal of the offending food, all or partial symptoms disappeared.

For those with only partial symptoms gone, chemical sensitivities were also suspected.

Hidden epidemics of the 90's

A New Field of Medicine

Most doctors have not yet received training in environmental medicine.

Without this training, doctors may not be able to correctly diagnose environmental illness.

Some doctors may even negate its existence.

In contrast, doctors trained in environmental medicine believe there may be a unsuspected epidemic of environmental illness.

Environmental illness results when a person's detoxification system becomes dysfunctional.

This happens when a person's system become overloaded from too many chemicals and/or nutrient deficiencies.

As a result, a person may adversely "react" to even small exposures to any chemical.

Symptoms from adverse reactions to chemicals may be almost anything.

Symptoms will vary depending upon the unique biochemistry of each individual and his or her present chemical load.

> *Examples of common symptoms of persons reacting to an environmental trigger are throat swelling, fatigue, respiratory problems, recurrent ear infections, muscular aches, chest pains, dizziness, and hyperactivity.*

Why Children Are More at Risk

Detoxifying enzymes are needed to break down toxic chemicals that have entered the body.

Children have lower levels of detoxifying enzymes.

Children have rapid cell division in order to grow.

Rapid cell division increases the probability of genetic mutations to subsequent generations of cells (which can initiate cancer).

Children under five breathe differently than other children and adults.

They have a faster respiratory rate in order to compensate for fewer and narrower branches in their respiratory tract.

Children inhale more toxins from the air, per pound of their body weight, than adults.

Children's playing habits and developmental exploration put them in closer contact with toxic chemicals.

Examples of such habits are crawling on a lawn or carpet recently sprayed with pesticides and putting plastic toys in the mouth.

Children have immature organs.

An example of such an organ is the brain, which continues to develop after birth.

The brain can be permanently affected by pesticides and other chemicals known to be neuro-toxins.

Avoiding the epidemic

Environmental illness is one of the most preventable illnesses around.

However, once a person does become sensitized to chemicals, it is an extremely difficult condition to reverse.

This is because initial exposures to the chemicals may have already caused permanent damage.

Therefore, to prevent environmental illness, one has to first believe in its existence.

Second, exposures to toxic chemicals intertwined in daily life need to be reduced and/or eliminated.

What if . . .

Your child has measles, but neither you or your doctor has knowledge of such an illness ?

What if your doctor incorrectly diagnoses the red bumps on your child's skin to be something else?

What if that something else requires a prescribed medication or surgery?

What if your child's condition does not improve with such treatment?

What if the condition does appear to improve, but new symptoms then occur?

What if, after numerous diagnoses and ineffective treatments to eliminate symptoms, you are told that your child really has a psychological problem?

But what if all this could have been avoided if you or your child's doctor knew how to recognize measles?

This analogy parallels a probable scenario for children reacting to environmental triggers, whose parents and doctors have no knowledge of environmental illness.

Ruling out environmental triggers

In some children, chronic conditions have been completely eliminated or greatly improved when environmental triggers were eliminated.

Such conditions are:

> **Asthma**
>
> **Bedwetting**
>
> **Colic**
>
> **Constipation**
>
> **Eczema**
>
> **Hyperactivity**
>
> **Learning problems**
>
> **Recurrent ear infections**
>
> **Recurrent sinus infections**
>
> **Recurrent bronchitis**
>
> **Recurrent diaper rash**
>
> **Stomach cramping**

Parents are encouraged to rule out environmental triggers as the cause of symptoms, negative behaviors, and/or chronic health conditions.

To do so, parents need to try and identify if a cause and effect relationship exists between symptoms and environmental exposures.

Since symptoms can be masked and/or do not always occur immediately after exposure, parents may need the assistance of a clinical ecologist.

Referral for a clinical ecologist in your area can be obtained from:

The American Academy of Environmental Medicine

P.O. Box 16106

Denver, Colorado 80216

On the Bedroom Walls

BASIC FACTS

A variety of formulas containing acrylics, synthetic rubber, and biocides (to retard mold) are used in latex paints.

Biocides may not be listed on product labels.

Wallpaper contains many toxic chemicals, not excluding pesticides and fungicides.

Vinyl and self-stick paper is considered to outgas more toxic chemicals than other wallpaper.

Wallpaper pastes also outgas toxic vapors.

CONCERNS

Over 700 toxic chemicals may be present in paint.

150 of these chemicals are thought to cause cancer.

Oil paints take months to become odorless since they contain petroleum solvents which outgas very slowly.

Persons in rooms painted with oil paints will then inhale these toxic vapors for months.

Persons in rooms that have been recently wallpapered will inhale toxic vapors.

Nontoxic Paints and Adhesives

SOLUTIONS

Purchase nontoxic paints and adhesives.

Reputable companies selling such products are:

AFM Enterprises
1440 Stacy Court
Riverside, CA 92507
(714) 781-6860
Free catalog

Livos Plantchemistry
1365 Rutina Circle
Santa Fe, NM 87501
(505) 438-3448
Free catalog

Sinan Company
P.O. Box 857
Davis, CA 95617
(916) 753-3104
Free catalog

The Natural Choice
Eco Design Co.
1365 Rufina Circle
Santa Fe, NM 87501

Carpet

BASIC FACTS

Chemicals in Carpet

In a chemical analysis of carpet, many hazardous chemicals were noted.

> *Examples of such chemicals are formaldehyde, benzene, and xylene (see glossary.)*

Hazardous chemicals are also used in carpet pads (e.g. polyurethane foam) as well as in carpet adhesives.

Even natural fiber rugs (e.g. cotton or wool) may be outgassing toxic chemicals.

Such rugs have probably been treated with a toxic dye or pesticide (for mothproofing).

Shampooing Carpets

Shampooing or steaming a carpet will not have any effect on the outgassing of new carpet.

Carpet chemicals are specifically designed to be water soluble.

Moreover, carpet shampoo may also have toxic ingredients such as sodium dodecylsulfate.

Old Carpet

Old carpet is a haven for microorganisms (molds, bacteria, yeast).

Studies have measured 10 million microorganisms per square foot of carpet.

Vacuuming only increases the number of microorganisms since it pulls them up from the padding to higher layers of carpet.

CONCERNS
Carpet Chemicals Linked to Symptoms and Cancer

Formaldehyde can cause *respiratory-tract irritation, chest tightness, headache,* and *fatigue.*

Benzene can cause cancer.

Xylene can cause *nausea, headaches,* and *vertigo.*

Sodium dodecylsufate is known to cause *eye and skin irritation, severe respiratory distress,* and *headaches.*

Allergies and Microorganisms

Many people develop allergies to the microorganisms (dustmites, mold, etc.) found in carpet.

Alternate Flooring

SOLUTIONS

Hardwood floors can be laid with nontoxic adhesives (see companies listed under Paints and Adhesives) or nailed to a subfloor.

Hardwood floors can be finished with *Crystal Shield,* a nontoxic finish, which can be purchased from:

> *Pace Industries*
>
> *710 Woodlawn Drive*
>
> *Thousand Oaks, CA 91360*
>
> *(805) 499-2911*

Pesticide-free wood can be purchased from:

Floyd Shelton Superior Floors
803 Jefferson Street
Wausau, WI 54401
1-800-247-4705, 715/842-5358

Ceramic tile can be laid with Portland cement. Tile can be purchased at local stores.

Bedroom Furniture

BASIC FACTS

Formaldehyde is used extensively in commercial furniture.

An otherwise empty home tripled its levels of formaldehyde after it was furnished.

Medium density fiberboard (which is used for dresser fronts and furniture tops) emits the highest levels of formaldehyde.

This is because medium density fiberboard has a higher resin to wood ratio.

Upholstered furniture can contain polyurethane foams, styrene foam chips, and foam rubber.

CONCERNS

In 1981, OSHA recommended that formaldehyde be handled as something potentially causing cancer in humans.

In 1987, the EPA concurred with this recommendation.

Polyurethane foam, styrene foam chips, and foam rubber all outgas harmful vapors.

Least Toxic Furniture

SOLUTIONS

Used and Unfinished Furniture

Purchase used furniture in order to reduce the outgassing associated with new furniture.

Buy unfinished furniture, and then use *Crystal Aire* to finish it.

Crystal Aire is a non-toxic sealant containing no petrochemicals or toxic ingredients.

Crystal Aire can be purchased from:

> *Pace Industries*
> *710 Woodlawn Drive*
> *Thousand Oaks, CA 91360*
> *(805) 496-6224*

Reupholstering

Existing furniture can be reupholstered by replacing foam rubber or synthetics with white cotton batting.

Slip covers can be made from untreated cotton, linen, or silk.

These materials can be purchased from:

The Cotton Place
P.O. Box 59721
Dallas, TX 75229
214/243-4149

Winter Silks
2700 Laura Lane
P.O. Box 130
Middleton, WI 53562
608/836-4600
800/648-7455

The Janice Corporation
198 Rt. 46
Budd Lake, NJ 07828
201/691-2979

Mattresses and Bedding

BASIC FACTS

THPC is commonly used as a flame retardant in mattresses.

THPC releases formaldehyde when fabric is wet (not an unusual occurance with a baby's mattress).

Polyurethane, which is also used in mattresses, releases toluene diisoyante.

Sheets and bedding are typically treated with additional formaldehyde (as compared to clothing).

This is done so that bedding does not need to be ironed, as well as to withhold numerous washings.

CONCERNS

Formaldehyde has been proven to cause cancer in animals and is suspected of doing so in humans.

Formaldehyde is also commonly known to cause respiratory tract irritation and acute dermatitis.

Toluene diisoyante can trigger serious pulmonary effects.

Untreated Mattresses and Bedding

SOLUTIONS

Purchase mattresses and bedding that has been untreated and made from natural fibers. Everything is made out of organically grown cotton and covered with unbleached, untreated cotton. Crib-size futon mattresses (as well as other sizes), innerspring mattresses, mattress pads, pillows, and comforters.

Such mattresses and bedding can be purchased from:

Dona Designs

825 Northlake Dr.

Richardson, TX 75080

(214) 235-0485

Free catalog

Pure Podunk, Inc.

Podunk Ridge Farm

RRI Box 69

Thetford Center, VT 05075

(802) 763-8651

Free catalog

Everything is made from untreated wool from sheep on a small
New England farm. Additionally, untreated cotton and linen
thread are used for covers. Offers crib-size futon mattresses
(as well as other sizes), comforters, mattress pads, and pillows

Seventh Generation

Colchester, VT 05446

(800) 456-1177

Free catalog

Unbleached and undyed bedding

The Bedroom Closet

BASIC FACTS

The closet may also be outgassing vapors from clothing of synthetic fibers (e.g. nylon, acrylic, and polyester) which are all made from petrochemicals.

According to NASA, polyester outgasses more than any other synthetic material.

Trichloroethylene may be outgassing from dry-cleaned clothing.

Formaldehyde may also be outgassing from permanent-press clothing.

Formaldehyde may also e outgassing from particle board (used in the interior of the closet).

CONCERNS

Trichloroethylene is suspected of causing cancer in humans.

Some symptoms associated with trichloroethylene are *gastrointestinal upsets, central nervous-system depression, heart and liver malfunctions, nausea, dizziness,* and *fatigue.*

Formaldehyde is suspected of causing cancer in humans.

Reducing Exposure from Closets

SOLUTIONS
Sealing Formaldehyde Vapors

Use *Crystal Aire,* a non-toxic sealant to seal in formaldehyde outgassing from particle board.

Crystal Aire can be purchased from:

> *Pace Industries*
>
> *710 Woodlawn Drive*
>
> *Thousand Oaks, CA 91360*
>
> *805/ 496-6224*

Clothing

Take dry-cleaned clothing out of plastic bags and hang to air out in the sun (if possible) for several days before placing in the closet.

Hang new synthetic and/or permanent press clothing in a closet other than the baby's room.

Natural Fiber Clothing

Reduce the amount of synthetic clothing outgassing from the closet by purchasing clothing made from natural fibers (e.g. cotton, wool).

Such clothing can be purchased in local stores as well as from:

After the Stork
1501 12th Street NW
Albuquerque, NM 87104
800/ 333-5437
Free catalog

The Natural Choice
Eco Design Co.
1365 Rufina Circle
Santa Fe, NM 87501
505/438-3448

Biobottoms
Box 6009
3820 Bodega Avenue
Petaluma, CA 94953
707/778-7945
Free catalog

Motherwear
P.O. Box 114
Northhampton, MA 01061
413/ 586-3488, also 584-8291
Free catalog

Toys

BASIC FACTS

Many toys are made from vinyl plastic, which includes polyvinylpyrrolidone (PVP).

Many toys also have polyvinyl chloride (PVC).

PVC releases vinyl chloride.

Plasticizers are used in PVC production.

Toys made from the mentioned materials are not required to carry warning labels.

Many of these toys are continually put into a baby's mouth.

CONCERNS

PVP is such a hazard that NASA has banned the use of it in space capsules.

PVP can cause cancer.   .

PVP can also cause a lung disease in which enlarged lymph nodes, lung masses, and changes in blood cells occur.

Vinyl chloride can cause cancer, birth defects, and mutations.

Vinyl chloride is on the EPA's list of 65 priority pollutants recognized as hazardous to human health.

Plasticizers can irritate the throat, mouth, and nose, as well as burn the skin.

Putting synthetic toys in the mouth provides an additional route for these toxic chemicals to enter the body.

If toys made from synthetic materials are kept in the nursery, they will outgas toxic vapors into the room.

These vapors will be subsequently inhaled throughout the night or any other time the baby is in the room.

Nontoxic Toys

SOLUTIONS

Store new plastic toys, as well as toys made from other synthetic materials, in a room different than your baby's.

Doing so will eliminate the outgassing of toxic vapors into your baby's room while he or she sleeps.

Purchase rattles, dolls, and toys made out of natural materials (e.g. wood, cotton) from local toy stores or from:

Baby Bunz and Company
P.O. Box 1717
Sebastopol, CA 95473
(707) 829-5347
Free catalog

Papa Don's Toys
Walker Creek Road
Walton, OR 97490
(503) 935-7604
Free catalog

Pure Podunk, Inc.
Podunk Ridge Farm
RR 1, Box 69
Thetford Center, VT 05075
(800) 776-3865
Free catalog

Northern Lights
P.O. Box 140
Milbridge, ME 04658
Free brochure

Air Fresheners & Deodorizers

BASIC FACTS

Air fresheners do not freshen the air of a room.

Air fresheners use chemicals to interfere with a person's ability to smell.

This is done by relying on a nerve-deadening agent or by coating nasal passages with an undetectable oil film.

Methoxychlor is a chlorinated hydrocarbon pesticide which is found in many common commercial deodorizers.

P-Dichlorobenzene and naphthalene are also toxic chemicals found in air fresheners.

CONCERNS

Methoxychlor accumulates in fat cells and overstimulates the central nervous system.

P-Dichlorobenzene and naphthalane are central nervous system depressants.

Naphthalene is a suspected human carcinogen.

Naphthalene can cause *headache, confusion, nausea,* and *urinary irritation.*

Nontoxic Air Fresheners

SOLUTIONS

Use sachets of herbs.

For diaper pails, use *Earth Care Odor Remover or Odor Fresh* in place of toxic deodorizers for diaper pails or other chemical air fresheners.

Earth Care Odor Remover or Odor Fresh are the trade names for zeolite.

Zeolite is a natural mineral that adsorbs bacteria and some indoor air contaminants.

Zeolite is completely nontoxic and inexpensive.

The Living Source
7005 Woodway Dr.
Waco, TX 76708
(817) 476-4878
Free catalog

Earth Care odor Remover can be purchased from:
Swanstar
Box 2596
Vista, CA 92085
619/945-1050

Odor Fresh can be purchased from:
The Living Source
7005 Woodway Dr.
Waco, TX 76708
817/776-4878

Products and information are available from:
Retail: Lotus Fulfillment Service
33719 116th St., NTB
Twin Lakes, WI 53181

Wholesale: Lotus Light
Box 1008, NTB
Silver Lake, WI 53170
414/889-8501

Cleaning Products

BASIC FACTS

The average American uses approximately 40 pounds of unsafe cleaning chemicals a year.

Not one single government agency is responsible for regulating or approving cleaning product formulations.

Cleaning products are not required by law to provide full disclosure labels (which list the product's entire ingredients).

Cleaning product labels are also not required to list which health hazards are associated with the chemicals used.

Common hazardous chemicals used in daily cleaning products are: *ammonia, benzene, chlorine, formaldehyde,* and *toluene.*

CONCERNS

Ammonia can cause *irritation of the eyes* and *respiratory tract.*

Benzene can cause *cancer* as well as *lightheadedness, disorientation,* and *fatigue.*

Chlorine can cause severe *respiratory-tract irritation, pulmonary edema,* and *skin rashes.*

Formaldehyde is suspected of causing cancer in humans.

Formaldehyde can also cause *swelling of the throat, watery eyes, respiratory problems, headaches,* and *asthma attacks.*

Toluene can cause *nervous system changes* and *irritability*, as well as *damage to the liver* and *kidneys*.

Nontoxic Cleaning Products

SOLUTIONS

Nontoxic cleaning products can be found in health food stores or purchased by mail order. Some reputable companies:

Ecover
4 Old Mill Rd.
P.O. Box 1140
Georgetown, CT 06829-1140

EcoSource
P.O.Box 1656
Sebastopol, CA 95473
(800) 274-7040

Granny's Old Fashioned
P.O. Box 256
Arcadia, CA 91006
(818) 577-1825
Free catalog

Mia Rose
1374 Logan, Unit C
Costa Mesa, CA 92626
(714) 662-5465, 800/292-6339
Free catalog

Real Goods Trading Corporation
966 Mazzoni St
Uriah, CA 95482
800/762-7325

Products and information are available from:
Retail: Lotus Fulfillment Service
33719 116th St., NTB
Twin Lakes, WI 53181

Wholesale: Lotus Light
Box 1008, NTB
Silver Lake, WI 53170

More Information

Read *Clean and Green,* by Anne Berthold-Bond; Ceres Publishing; P.O. Box 87; Woodstock, NY 12498.

> *Clean and Green is an excellent, easy-to-read book with countless nontoxic alternatives and home-made recipes for toxic commercial products.*

Pest Control

BASIC FACTS

Organophosphates

Organophosphates are a specific group of pesticides which are which are routinely used.

Organophosphates originated out of chemical warfare research.

Organophosphates are derived from the same family of chemicals used to make nerve gas.

Neurotoxins

Pesticides are neurotoxins (chemicals which affect the brain and nervous system).

Symptoms

Symptoms may not appear immediately following exposure.

This is because pesticides can be stored in body tissues.

Small amounts of stored pesticides can be slowly released into the bloodstream over a period of months.

EPA Registration

EPA registration is not synonymous with pesticide safety.

According to the Code of Federal Regulations, CFR 162.10(a)(5), it is a violation of labeling requirements to claim that pesticides are safe.

Lack of federal funding to enforce this code makes it easy for manufacturers to continue to make false safety claims.

Chemlawn, one of the nation's largest pest control companies, claimed their products were "practically non-toxic" and "do not present a health risk."

State Attorney General Robert Abrams of New York recently filed suit against this claim and won.

Before 1977 pesticides were allowed to be registered without testing.

All pesticides registered prior to that date are still allowed on the market today.

After 1977, a pesticide could be registered if its perceived benefits outweighed the known risks in the very limited testing done.

Inert Ingredients

Pesticide inert ingredients can comprise as much as 90-99% of the total product.

Inert ingredients are not required to be listed on product labels.

Of the approximate 1200 inert ingredients used, there is virtually no information available for 800 of them.

55 inert ingredients have already been established to be hazardous toxins.

Even though DDT has been banned since the seventies, an EPA staff member has confirmed that DDT is listed as an inert (secret) ingredient in numerous currently used registered pesticides.

Secret inert ingredients in pesticide formulations makes it impossible to accurately claim a product's safety.

Industry Sponsored Testing and Research

Due to a lack of funds, the EPA and FDA must rely heavily on industry-sponsored testing and research to determine health risks associated with pesticides.

CONCERNS
Falsified Studies

Industry-sponsored research and testing may result in falsified reports.

This was proven true in 1981 when the owners of Industrial Biotest Labs were convicted for fraudulent testing.

The owners were sent to prison for falsifying 90% of more than 2,000 pesticide studies submitted to the EPA.

As of mid 1984, less than 243 of these studies were replaced.

The EPA has now decided to let the remainder wait to go through the normal process of review.

Due to continual cutbacks in budget, this not likely to happen until sometime in the far future.

Therefore, the majority of the products whose registrations were issued based on Biotest's fraudulent testing still remain on the market today.

Consumers do not have knowledge which products contain pesticides that were in the falsified reports.

Untested Pesticides

Consumers are also exposed to additional untested pesticides when they used product formulations with pesticides registered before 1977.

False Security

Persons may falsely believe they are not being affected by pesticides.

This is because they may not have knowledge of how pesticides are stored in the body.

They may not also know of the long term affects (e.g sterility, birth defects) which have been associated with pesticides.

Effects on Children's Brain

Pesticides, which are neurotoxins, can easily pass into the brain, a lipid organ.

A child's brain is likely to be more affected by pesticides than an adult.

This is because a child's brain is still developing after birth.

Nontoxic Pest Control

SOLUTIONS

NonToxic Services

To control the pests in your home, employ a company using non-toxic formulas.

Be suspicious of any company that tells you their product is non-toxic, but still requires you to leave the home for several hours.

Also be suspicious if any smell lingers after application.

Reputable companies offering nontoxic services are:

Flea Busters/ Rx for Fleas

1-800-666-3532 (for referral of Flea Buster distributorship in your area. Located in Alabama, California, Connecticut, Delaware, Florida, Georgia, Hawaii, Louisiana, Maryland, New Jersey, North Carolina, Ohio, Oregon, South Carolina, Texas, Washington (state), Washington, D.C.)

Flea Buster's nontoxic formula is applied by a serviceman and is guaranteed for one year. The product is EPA registered.

Non-toxic Termite Control

1-800-543-5651

The above number is the corporate office number of Etex Ltd. Upon calling it, a person will refer you to a local, licensed pest control company in your area that uses a completely non-toxic approach to eliminate termites. This approach is also effective against powderpost beetles.

By Yourself

Control pests using nontoxic products found in health food stores or ordered from:

Mia Rose

1374 Logan, Unit C

Costa Mesa, CA 92626

(714) 666-5465

Free catalog

Natural ingredients in a product called Air Therapy act as an effective repellant against pests (as well being a general air freshener).

Safer, Inc.

189 Wells Avenue

Newton, MA 02159

Offers a wide variety of non-toxic products for controlling pests.

Products and information are available from:

Retail: Lotus Fulfillment Service	*Wholesale: Lotus Light*
33719 116th St., NTB	*Box 1008, NTB*
Twin Lakes, WI 53181	*Silver Lake, WI 53170*
	414/889-8501

More Information

Read *Pest Control You Can Live With* by Debra Graff

(Earth Stewardship Press; P.O. Box 1316; Sterling, VA 22170).

This book is an inexpensive, simple book with clear instructions for nontoxic control of common household pests.

Disposable Diapers

BASIC FACTS

Time in Diapers

A baby spends approximately 20,000 hours in diapers.

History of Disposables

Disposable diapers have only been on the market since the early sixties.

Disposables used to be fatter and wadded with more paper fluff to keep babies dry.

Today disposables are slimmer and more heavily doused with superabsorbent chemicals.

Long term effects from exposure to these diapers are unknown.

Chemicals in Diapers

Sodium polyacrylate is a superabsorbent chemical found in a disposable diaper's paper pulp.

Dyes are used in disposable diapers.

Polyethylene is used in disposable diapers.

Fragrances are used in disposable diapers.

Disposables diapers have been bleached white in a process which includes the chemical dioxin.

Little is known about the amounts of dioxin transferred to a baby via disposables.

Diaper Rash

In a study in the Journal of Pediatrics, 54% of the infants wearing disposables had rashes.

This compared to only 18% of infants wearing cloth diapers having rashes.

The study cited several reasons for more rashes among babies wearing disposable diapers.

One reasons attributed allergic reactions to the chemicals used in disposables.

Other reasons were attributed to lack of air, higher temperatures, and the probability that disposables were changed less often.

Waste from Disposables

Baby excrement carries more than 100 intestinal viruses.

Approximately 5 million tons of untreated waste is brought to landfills via disposables.

Untreated waste may contribute to ground water contamination.

Untreated waste may also attract flies and other airborne insects which carry and transmit diseases.

CONCERNS

Health Effects of Chemicals in Diapers

Sodium polyacrylate has been reported in pediatric journals as sticking to babies' genitals and passing through urine.

Dyes, are known to damage the *central nervous system, kidneys,* and *liver.*

Polyethylene is suspected of causing cancer in humans.

Symptoms reported to the FDA related to fragrances are (but not limited to) *headaches, dizziness,* and *rashes.*

Dioxin in Diapers

Dioxin is known to migrate from paper products through the skin.

Small residues of dioxin may remain on disposables.

These residues may come in direct contact with a baby's skin.

In the smallest detectable quantities, dioxin has been known to cause *liver disease, immune system depression,* and *genetic damage* in laboratory animals.

According to the EPA, dioxin is the most toxic of all cancer-linked chemicals.

General Public Health

Disposable diapers present a general public health concern since their contents often contain contagious viruses.

Viruses from the fecal matter of babies is of particular concern.

This is because babies are usually vaccinated with live vaccines.

Nontoxic Diapering

SOLUTIONS

Diapering with Cloth

The cloth diaper is slipped inside a diaper cover made from natural materials.

The diaper cover is then secured with adjustable velcro closures.

With this method, cloth diapering takes about 10 seconds.

Diaper Covers

Nikkys are a popular brand of breathable diaper covers.

Nikkys are made from natural materials (cotton and wool) which require no pins.

Bumpkins, advertised as a all-in-one-washable cloth diaper, is another popular brand name.

Disposable Non-Plastic Diapers

The *Dovetail*, which is made from wood pulp and biodegrades in one month, is a new disposable, non-toxic diaper.

The *Dovetail* is used with a diaper cover as with cloth diapers.

Companies

These alternatives to disposable diapers can be purchased from:

Baby Bunz and Company
P.O. Box 1717
Sebastopol, CA 95473
(707) 829-5347
Free catalog

Biobottoms
Box 6009
3820 Bodega Avenue
Petaluma, CA 94953
(707) 778-7945

Family Clubhouse
6 Chiles Avenue
Asheville, NC 28803
800 - 876 -1574
Free catalog

Motherwear
P.O. Box 114
Northhampton, MA 01061
(413) 586-3488
Free catalog

Diaper Services

Diaper services can be used to clean cloth diapers.

It is approximately 500 dollars cheaper to use cloth diapers with a diaper service than using disposable diapers.

The toll-free number for assistance in finding a diaper service near you (if none are listed in the phone book) is 800 - 462-6237 .

Soothing Baby's Skin

BASIC FACTS

BHT/BHA are two common ingredients found in products designed to soothe a baby's skin.

Talc is a common ingredient found in most baby powders.

CONCERNS

BHA is suspected of causing cancer in humans.

BHT is known to cause *metabolic stress, depression* of *growth rate,* and *liver damage.*

BHT is also known to cause cancer in animals.

Talc may be contaminated with carcinogenic asbestos fibers.

Nontoxic
Soothing & Cleaning Products

SOLUTIONS

Dioxin-free, no alcohol, no artificially-scented baby wipes are offered by:
Seventh Generation
Colchester, VT 05446
(800) 456-1177

Talc-free baby powder is offered by

Autumn Harp	*Natural Lifestyle Supplies*
28 Rockydale Road	*16 Lookout Drive*
Bristol, VT 05443	*Asheville, NC 28804*
(802) 453 - 4807	*(800) 752 -2775*

Petroleum-free jelly is offered by:

Autumn Harp

(See address listed on preceding card)

Motherwear

P.O. Box 114

Northhampton, MA 01061

(413) 586-3488, also 584-8291

Products and information are available from:

Retail: Lotus Fulfillment Service

33719 116th St., NTB

Twin Lakes, WI 53181

Wholesale: Lotus Light

Box 1008, NTB

Silver Lake, WI 53170

414/889-8501

Laundry Detergent

BASIC FACTS

Manufacturers are not required to list the exact ingredients on laundry product labels.

This is legal because legislation protects trade secrecy.

Warnings on product labels only refer to immediate, acute effects (e.g if swallowed).

Long-term effects associated with many chemicals used in laundry detergent formulas are never mentioned.

Many laundry detergents have *ammonia, ethanol, fragrances, naphthalene, phenol,* and *sodium alluminosillicate.*

CONCERNS

Ammonia is known to cause *skin burning* and *irritation to the eyes* and *respiratory tract*.

Ethanol is known to depress the central nervous system.

Ethanol can also cause *nausea, vertigo, impaired motor coordination,* and *drowsiness.*

Synthetic fragrances have been known to cause a long list of symptoms, including *hyperactivity, irritability,* and other *behavior changes.*

Naphthalene is suspected of causing cancer in humans.

Naphthalene has also been associated with *skin irritation, headache,* and *confusion.*

Phenol is suspected of causing cancer in humans.

Phenol has also been known to cause *skin eruptions, skin peeling, swelling, hives* and *burning.*

Sodium aluminosillicate is also sometimes used as a pesticide.

Nontoxic Laundry Detergents

SOLUTIONS

Reputable non-toxic laundry detergents are:

Ecover Liquid Laundry
Mercantile Food Company
4 Old Mill Road
P.O. Box 1140
Georgetown, CT 06829

Life Tree Premium Laundry Liquid
Sunrise Lane
780 Greenwich Street
New York NY 10014
(212) 242 - 7014
Free catalog

Granny's Power Plus Laundry
Concentrate
Granny's Old Fashioned Products
P.O. Box 256
Arcadia, CA 91006
(818) 577 - 1825
Free catalog

EcoSource Laundry Detergent
Concentrate
EcoSource
P.O. Box 1656
Sebastopol, CA 95473
(800)274-7040
Free catalog

Bleach

BASIC FACTS

Ingredients found in bleach include chlorine, lye, artificial dyes, and synthetic fragrances.

Many people report adverse reactions to chlorine residues left in clothing that has been laundered.

CONCERNS

Toxicology books report that chlorine is "toxic as a skin irritant and by inhalation."

Chlorine, lye, artificial dyes, and synthetic fragrances are believed to be hazardous to human health by many experts.

Nontoxic Bleach

SOLUTIONS

Bleach, without chlorine and other toxic chemicals, can be substituted for traditional commercial products.

Such products are:

Ecover Alternative Bleach
Mercantile Food Company
4 Old Mill Road
P.O. Box 1140
Georgetown, CT 06829

WinterWhite Powdered Bleach
Sunrise Lane
780 Greenwich Street
New York, NY 10014
212/ 242 - 7014

Soap

BASIC FACTS

Soap manufacturers are not required to list ingredients.

Ingredients known to be in soaps are *ammonia, BHA, BHT, colors, formaldehyde, fragrance, glycols,* and *phenol.*

CONCERNS

Fragrances in soap have been known to cause *dry skin, redness,* and *rashes.*

Ammonia, BHA, BHT, colors, formaldehyde, glycols, and *phenol* have all been associated with significant health concerns.

Nontoxic Soap

SOLUTIONS

Reputable non-toxic, natural soaps manufactured and found in most health food stores from:

Dr. Bronner's

All-One-God-Faith, Inc.

Escondido, CA 92015

Desert Essence

9510 Basser Ave, #A

Chatsworth, CA 91311

818/709-5900

Weleda

P.O. Box 769

Spring Valley, NY 10977

914/ 352 - 6145

Light Mountain Soap

by Lotus Brands

Box 325

Twin Lakes, WI 53181

414/ 889-8561

Products and information are available from:

Retail: Lotus Fulfillment Service   *Wholesale: Lotus Light*
33719 116th St., NTB   *Box 1008, NTB*
Twin Lakes, WI 53181   *Silver Lake, WI 53170*
                                       414/889-8501

Shampoo

BASIC FACTS

Some ingredients found in shampoos are *ammonia, colors, cresol, EDTA, ethanol, formaldehyde, fragrances, nitrates/nitrosamines, PVP,* and *sulfur compounds.*

Cosmetic products are not required to be tested for safety by any government agency.

Cosmetic manufacturers are not required to list all ingredients on product labels.

The FDA can only intervene after a product has been on the market.

To do so, there has to be enough significant evidence to present in court.

CONCERNS

Ammonia, colors, cresol, EDTA, ethanol, formaldehyde, fragrances, nitrates/nitrosamines, PVP, and *sulfur compounds* have all been linked to symptoms and adverse health conditions.

Consumers are using products which have not passed any government testing.

Consumers are using products without knowledge of their actual ingredients.

Nontoxic Shampoo

SOLUTIONS

Reputable nontoxic baby shampoos are manufactured or distributed by:

Aubrey Organics
4419 N. Manhattan Avenue
Tampa, FL 33614
(818) 876 - 4878
Found in most health food stores

Tom's of Maine
Seventh Generation
Colchester, VT 05446
(800) 456-1177
Found in most health food stores

Autumn Harp
28 Rockydale Road
Bristol, VT 05443
(802) 453 - 4807
Found in most health food stores

Products and information are available from:

Retail: Lotus Fulfillment Service
33719 116th St., NTB
Twin Lakes, WI 53181

Wholesale: Lotus Light
Box 1008, NTB
Silver Lake, WI 53170
414/889-8501

Pesticides in Food

BASIC FACTS
Removing Pesticides

In most cases, washing produce will not eliminate pesticide residues.

This is because many pesticides are systemic.

Most pesticides are also formulated to be water resistant.

Waxing and Pesticides

The common practice of waxing produce actually seals in pesticides residues.

Additionally, a fungicide is added to the wax.

Pesticide Residue Limits

The theoretical legal pesticide residue limits are based on an 125 pound adult.

The limits assume that a person is only exposed to one pesticide - and never more than one simultaneously.

The "safe pesticide residue standards" were made in the sixties and have not been updated.

These standards also do not reflect the increased consumption of produce over the past decades.

Examples:

Within this EPA's safe level, a person can eat no more than a half a pound per year of artichokes, avocados, blueberries, cantaloupe, honeydew melon, eggplant, plums, tangerines, nectarines, or radishes.

Anyone eating more than this is potentially exposed to more pesticide residues than what even the agency considers to be safe.

Number of Pesticides Applied

Non-organic fruit and vegetables have multiple numbers of pesticide residue.

Examples:

More than 100 different chemicals are commonly used on tomatoes.

75 different chemicals are commonly used on cucumbers.

50-60 different chemicals are commonly used on carrots and lettuce.

Imported Food

Imported food has food has almost double the amount of pesticides than domestically grown food.

Commonly, these pesticides are those which are unregistered, banned, or severely restricted in the United States.

U.S. law allows manufacturers in this country to still make these pesticides, as long as they are for export.

Pesticides Registered Before 1977

All pesticides registered before 1977 are still currently used on food crops.

None of these pesticides have been tested for cancer, birth defects, or chromosome damage.

This is because they were registered prior to the EPA mandate to test chemicals for health hazards.

Inspection

The FDA inspects less than 1% of the food that is sold in grocery stores.

More than half of the pesticides used on food crops cannot be detected by routine laboratory methods.

Certified Organic vs. Pesticide-free

Certified organic food may be very different than food labeled "pesticide-free."

Pesticide-free food may just mean that no pesticides were detected at a random sample at the dock.

CONCERNS
Health Problems

Numerous studies have linked pesticides to cancer, birth defects, genetic defects, and neurological effects.

Food with Illegal Pesticides

Up to 70% of the food grown abroad with unregistered, banned, or severely restricted pesticides is then exported back to this country.

This food is then sold in local supermarkets.

Overlooked Key Points

The "safe" limits do not take in account children of lesser weight or the specific dietary habits of children.

The "safe" limits do not take in account the increase of produce consumption of persons living in the 90's.

Even though multiple pesticides are routinely applied to one crop, present testing does not include the health effect of the total number of pesticides per fruit or vegetable.

Foods with Untested Pesticides

Consumers are eating foods that have been sprayed with pesticides that have never been tested.

Problems with Pesticide-free Food (vs. Certified Organic)

Since more than half the pesticides applied on crops cannot be detected with routine methods, it is possible that "pesticide-free" food actually does have pesticide residues.

"Pesticide-free" food can also be contaminated further down the line, past inspection at the docks.

ELIMINATING AND/OR REDUCING PESTICIDES FROM FOOD
SOLUTIONS
Organic Food

Buy organic food whenever possible.

If organic food is not available locally, it can be ordered by mail.

Most companies ship their perishables in a styro-insulated box with ice packs in order to ensure proper refrigeration.

Mail order companies with organic food are as follows:

Gold Mine Natural Food Co.
1947 30th Street
San Diego, CA 92102
800/475-3663., 619/234-9711

Green Earth Natural Foods
2545 Prairie Avenue
Evanston, IL 60201
708/864-8949

Mountain Ark Trading Co.
1601 Pump Station Rd., Box 3170
Fayetteville, AR 72701
800/ 643-8909

Perlinger Naturals
238 Petaluma Ave.
Sebastopol, CA 95472
707/ 829-8363
(Baby food)

Organic Foods Express
11003 Emack Rd.
Beltsville, MD 20705
301/816-4944

Walnut Acres
Penns Creek, PA 17862
717/ 837-0601

A manufacturer of organic baby foods which are available in natural food stores nationwide:

> Earth's Best Baby Food
> PO Box 887
> Middleburg, VT 05753
> 802/388-7974, 800/442-4221

Currently the term "organic" is legally defined in only 3 states.

In California, organic is defined as food that is *"produced, harvested, distributed, stored, processed, and packaged without the application of synthetically compounded fertilizers, pesticides, or growth regulators."*

Precautions With Non-organic Food

When purchasing non-organic food, buy domestically grown food (versus imported food).

If necessary, ask your grocery to label food accordingly.

Beware of cosmetically perfect or out-of-season fruit.

More pesticides have probably been used to make the fruit look so perfect or to be available during the off-season.

Note that peeling fruits and vegetables (sprayed with pesticides) may remove some pesticide residues, but not if a systemic pesticide has been used.

Note that the following produce are routinely waxed: *apples, avocados, bell peppers, cantaloupes, cucumbers, eggplants, grapefruits, lemons, limes, melons, oranges, parsnips, passion fruits, peaches, pineapples, pumpkins, rutabagas, squashes, sweet potatoes, tomatoes, and turnips.*

Note which foods have been identified as having more pesticide residues and carcinogenic chemicals in comparison to other foods.

Example:

David Steinman, author of Diet for a Poisoned Planet, has classified some foods as red and yellow light.

A red light label indicates the food is unsafe to eat at all times.

This is due to the high number of pesticide residues found and types of carcinogenic pesticides used on the crop.

According to Steinman, red light foods are non-organic raisins and peanuts.

Yellow light foods are considered to be almost as harmful as red light foods.

According to Steinman, yellow light foods are non-organic: apricots, apples, blackberries, blueberries, cantaloupe, cherries, cranberries, grapes, honeydews, nectarines, peaches, pears, plums, prunes, strawberries, artichokes, broccoli, celery, tomatoes, cucumbers, bell peppers, lettuce, potatoes, spinach, string beans, squash, and tomatoes.

More Information

Read *Pesticide Alert*, by Lawrie Mott and Karen Snyder.

Pesticide Alert is a short, easy-to-read book that explains specifically which pesticides are used in which foods.

Meat, Pork & Poultry

BASIC FACTS

Pesticides in Food

Pesticides are used to grow animal feed.

Pesticides bioaccumulate up the food chain.

Meat has 14x more pesticide residues than produce.

Cancer in Chickens

The Surgeon General estimates that over 90% of all commercial chickens are infected with leukosis.

Leukosis is a viral cancer which is peculiar to chickens.

Chickens, with leukosis, are allowed to go to market if they do not "look too repugnant."
The tumors on these chickens are cut away before the chickens are sold.

Artificial colors are then be used to make the chicken look healthy.

Salmonella in Chicken

As reported in Newsweek magazine, over 1/3 of all the chicken in the U.S. have salmonella.

Testing

U.S.D.A. inspectors are now allowed approximately 3 seconds to examine a carcass.

For toxic residues, the U.S.D.A. only tests one out of every quarter million slaughtered animals.

This test is only capable of detecting less than 10% of the toxic chemicals known to be used with animals.

CONCERNS

Salmonella poisoning is usually mistaken for the flu, as symptoms are very similar.

Consumers are eating meat and poultry which most likely has not been tested for toxic chemicals.

Consumers are purchasing chicken which comes from diseased animals.

Consumers may not be aware that they are ingesting a higher number pesticide residues (than found in produce) when they consume meat and poultry.

Avoiding Contaminated Meat, Pork & Poultry

SOLUTIONS

Changes in Diet

Reduce the amount of meat, pork, and poultry eaten.

Adding more organic whole grains (e.g. rice, barley, oats) to your baby's diet.

Organic Meat and Poultry

Purchase meat, pork, and poultry that comes from animals who have only been fed organic grains.

Mail order companies which sell such meat, pork, and poultry are:

Green Earth Natural Foods
2545 Prairie Avenue
Evanston, IL 60201
708)864-8949

Natural Beef Farms Food Distribution
4399-A Henniger Ct.
Chantilly, VA 22021
(703) 631-0881

Reducing the Risk of Salmonella Poisoning

Pack raw meat and poultry separate from other grocery items in the cart and bag (to prevent from dripping on other food).

Refrigerate as soon as possible.

Thaw meat in the refrigerator versus room temperature.

Wash hands and utensils immediately after handling raw meat or poultry.

Cook thoroughly.

Antibiotics and Growth Hormones in Meat & Poultry

BASIC FACTS

Increase in Antibiotics

Routine administration of antibiotics to livestock has increased by 400% in the last 20 years.

New Bacteria

The widespread use of antibiotics may actually generate new species of bacteria.

This is because bacteria can become resistant to antibiotics which are given regularly.

The use of antibiotics has not proven successful in eliminating all microbial contamination.

In the last decade, bacterial contamination of poultry has increased in spite of the increase in antibiotics.

The Effects of Hormones on Children

In the Journal of Puerto Rico Medical Association, Dr. Carmen Sanchez published the results of a study on children (as young as four and five years old).

These children had premature puberty symptoms (e.g. almost fully developed breasts, pubic hair).

The study stated that the children's premature puberty symptoms were the result of their consumption of local whole milk, poultry, and beef.

The study reported that the children's symptoms specifically resulted from the hormones administered to the animals.

In most cases, when the children were taken off the milk, poultry, and beef, their symptoms regressed.

DES and Other Growth Hormones

DES is a growth hormone which has been banned because of its direct link to cancer.

DES was still found to be illegally implanted in one half million cattle since the FDA ruling.

Other sex hormones (some which contain substances of DES) are presently routinely administered and legal to use.

CONCERNS
Health Effects

Regularly ingesting animals or products from animals given antibiotics may have serious consequences.

They may make these drugs ineffective for persons needing them in life-threatening situations.

This is because toxic bacteria easily becomes immune to antibiotics given to humans, also.

Regular ingestion may also prompt mild to severe allergic reactions in some individuals.

Banned in Other Countries

In 1984, the EEC (the European Economic Community) passed a ruling on 11 United States major meat producers.

The ruling declared these companies ineligible for exporting their products to the Common Market.

This was due to its concern over health hazards associated with hormones given to animals.

There is no restriction on these companies in the United States.

Meat & Poultry Without Antibiotics and Growth Hormones

SOLUTIONS

Kosher meat and chicken have no antibiotics or growth hormones.

Organic meat and poultry also have no antibiotics or growth hormones. (See address for such companies under Organic Meat, Pork, and Poultry.)

Local health food and other stores may carry meat and poultry labeled as "natural."

A natural label generally means that the animal was given no antibiotics or growth hormones.

Note that a "natural" label does not necessarily indicate that the animals were given organic feed.

If not fed organic feed, natural meat or poultry will still have pesticide residues, even though the hormone and antibiotic exposures have been eliminated.

Food Additives

BASIC FACTS

Food Additive Statistics

The average American eats approximately 150 pounds of additives each year.

More than 3,000 different additives are now intentionally used in processed food.

Industry experts predict that this number will double during the next decade.

Colors

Most colors used in food are considered to be very harmful by leading experts in this field.

The use of colors in food has increased elevenfold since 1940.

Food Additive Testing

Responsibility for testing of additives is done by the manufacturer.

Such testing is very limited and does not include the synergistic effect.

The synergistic effect is what might happen when one or more additives are consumed together.

The Approved "GRAS" List

Some additives are exempted from any testing if they have been "prior sanctioned" or seem to be safe.

These additives are labeled GRAS ("generally recognized as safe") and can be used without any limit.

Since 1949, the FDA has had to ban at least two dozen widely used additives which were once on the approved list.

Modified Starch

Modified starch is a common additive found in baby food.

CONCERNS
Children and Food Additives

Children are more susceptible to health hazards associated with food additives.

This is because a child's central nervous system is still developing.

In some children, a number of additives are believed to cause *allergic reactions, cancer, heart disease, brain damage, learning disorders,* and *hyperactivity* .

Despite both studies and warnings from experts in the field, colors are still used in countless food products on the market.

The Problem GRAS Classification

The GRAS classification does not guarantee safety since many of these additives have been subsequently banned outright or removed from the GRAS list.

Such examples are cyclamates, saccharin, saffrole, brominated vegetable oil, and many artificial colors.

The Problem with Modified Starch

The concern with modified starch used in baby food is related to the chemicals used to manufacture the starch.

These chemicals have been linked to heart, kidney, and intestinal disorders.

Reducing Food Additives and Eliminating Harmful Ones

SOLUTIONS

Less Processed Food

Reduce the amount of processed foods eaten by your child.

This will automatically reduce the amount of food additives ingested by your child.

Recognizing Additives

Become familiar with food additives listed on labels.

Know what studies and risks have been associated with them with food studies, and then buy food accordingly.

> Note that Blue No. 1, Blue No.2, Green No. 3, Red No 3, Red No. 40, Yellow No 5, Orange B, and Citrus Red No. 2 are recommended to be avoided at all times by leading experts in this field.

Note that foods which are typically artificially colored are: sweet potatoes, marachino cherries, ice cream, cake, candy, frosting, fillings, butter, oleomargarine, cheese, bologna, hot dogs, soft drinks, oranges, gelatin, and sausage.

Note that brominated vegetable oil (BVO), butylated hydroxytoluene (BHT), sodium nitrate, sodium nitrate, butylated hydroxyanisole (BHA), saccharin, MSG, and nutrasweet have also been recommended to be avoided by many leading experts.

Milk

BASIC FACTS
Bacteria in Milk

Bacteria can originate from fecal matter that has contaminated the cow's udder and teats.

This contamination is not required to be completely removed with pasteurization.

By government standards, bacteria must be kept at a minimum, but milk is not required to be sterile.

Dairy Products and Pesticides

No milk or dairy products sold in the U.S. (unless it came from cows that were fed organic feed) is without pesticide residues.

Milk has 5 1/2 times more pesticide residues than produce.

In a sampling of cow's milk, the residues of toxic chemicals were detected.

96% of the sampling had dieldrin; 93% had heptachlor epoxide; 73% had lindane; 67% had chlordane, and 48% had DDT.

Antibiotics in Milk

Sulfamethazine is an antibiotic added to animal feed in order to prevent respiratory illness.

Sulfamethazine is believed to be a cancer-causing and allergenic drug.

It is banned for use in milk-producing animals.

Even still, residues of this drug were found in 73% of the milk samples taken in ten major American cities in 1988.

Milk Advertisements

Commercials about milk are not public service announcements.

They are commercials to promote milk sales.

The American dairy farmers are willing to tax themselves to promote milk sales.

This is because they found that every 15 cents taxed brings back a return of $1.68 in new revenues.

Milk and Allergy

Milk has been named as one of the leading sources of food allergy in children.

Milk has also been associated with recurrent ear infections.

CONCERNS

Parents may have been led to believe that milk is "the perfect, healthy drink" for all children.

Parents may not be aware that pesticides, antibiotics, and hormones are found in milk today.

Dairy products may not be suspected as a possible cause of recurrent symptoms (e.g. ear infections, runny nose, etc.) by most parents and doctors.

Reducing Exposures to Dairy Product Contaminants

SOLUTIONS
Diet Changes

Reduce the amount of milk and diary products given to your child.

Purchase alternate products such as soy cheese, soy milk, rice milk, and almond milk (which can be found in health food stores).

Note foods which are high in calcium (e.g. broccoli, almonds, and kale) to supplement your child's diet when reducing dairy products.

More Information

Read *Don't Drink Your Milk*, by pediatrician Dr. Frank Oski.

Don't Drink Your Milk offers a well-supported, opposing view to the traditional recommendation of drinking 3 glasses a milk a day.

Breast Milk

BASIC FACTS

How Breast Milk Becomes Contaminated

Breast milk can become contaminated from chemicals stored in a mother's body.

These chemicals represent a mother's past and present exposures to toxins, which have bioaccumulated in her body.

During breastfeeding, the stored chemicals are released into the breast milk.

Chemicals in Breast Milk

According to the EPA, the average American breastfed infant ingests 10 times the FDA's maximum allowable intake of the toxic chemical PCB.

In doses as small as a few parts per billion, PCB causes cancer and birth defects in test animals.

DDT has been banned since the seventies, yet there is still no downward trend of DDT in sampled breast milk.

Premature Infants

Premature infants are more vulnerable to contaminated breast milk because they tend to have impaired elimination mechanisms.

The blood brain barrier of premature infants may also be more easily breached.

Formula

Any alternative (formula) to breastfeeding is also going to be contaminated.

Breast Milk of Vegetarian Mothers

Studies have shown that the breast milk of vegetarian mothers to be very different than non-vegetarian mothers.

Vegetarian mothers' milk contained only 1 - 2% of the pesticides found in samples of milk of non-vegetarian mothers.

CONCERNS

Mothers may not be aware that exposures to chemicals in food and the environment may contaminate their breast milk.

Mothers may not be aware that quick weight loss diets may increase the risk of breast milk contamination since dieting mobilizes fat (where toxins are stored).

Reducing Breast Milk Contamination

SOLUTIONS
General Recommendations

While breast milk may be contaminated, it is still considered by all authorities to be the preferred choice for infants.

This is because the nutritional, immunological, and psychological benefits of breastfeeding outweigh the environmental risks.

A soy formula is recommended for babies who are not going to be breastfed.

Less Contaminated Breastmilk

The La Leche League International makes the following recommendation to reduce breast milk contamination:

Reduce the amount of dairy and meat products eaten.

Avoid foods with fat.

Avoid quick weight-loss.

Reduce a mother's overall exposures to pesticides.

A more conservative recommendation (in addition to avoiding foods with fat and quick weight-loss) would be as follows:

Completely eliminate meat and dairy products (unless they came from animals that had only been fed organic feed).

Completely eliminate all exposures to pesticides, including commercial food sprayed with these chemicals.

Water

BASIC FACTS
Increased Chlorine in Water

Chlorine has been added to our water as a disinfectant.

The need for chlorine in our water supply has increased due to the spread of nitrates and phosphates from agriculture run-off.

As an example, Chicago has increased the amount of chlorine in the water supply by over 75% in the last 30 years.

Cancer-causing Agents in Water

A laboratory of the EPA has found two cancer-causing agents to form in water when chlorine interacts with humus (organic matter from the decay of plants).

One of these agents is called MX.

MX has shown up in every water sample.

MX is believed to induce genetic mutations.

The other agent is DCA.

DCA is another mutagen and can also cause live cancers.

Water Contamination

Water can become contaminated from bacteria and viruses.

Water can become contaminated from inorganic matter (e.g. asbestos, lead, nitrates).

Water can become contaminated from organic chemicals (e.g. pesticides, herbicides, vinyl chloride).

The EPA has identified more than 700 regularly occurring contaminants in water.

Twenty-two of these chemicals are already known to cause cancer.

The EPA regularly monitors just 8 inorganic chemicals and 10 organic chemicals found in water.

Contaminants from Water Pipes

Lead, asbestos, and copper are common contaminants from water pipes.

This is why water reports from the municipal site might be very different than actual water found in the home.

Lead in Water

The EPA estimates that 25% of a child's lead intake still comes from drinking water.

This statistic is as high as 40-60% for infants.

Lead is now thought to be a serious health hazard at even lower levels than originally stated as dangerous.

Some symptoms of lead poisoning are *neurological damage, impaired hearing,* and *impaired function of blood cells.*

Others may have no or non-specific symptoms such as *headaches, muscle aches,* and *rashes.*

Because the Center of Diseases now believes lead poisoning to be such a widespread problem, it makes the following recommendation:

> *All children between the ages of 6 months and 6 years should have a blood test for lead.*

Bottled Water

Bottled water is not required by law to be pure.

Note that legally, "bottled water" is just that - water in bottle.

Water, bottled in plastic containers, may become contaminated from the container.

This is because the plastic can leach right into the water.

This is especially true of water that has been bottled and sitting on shelves for long periods of time before being consumed.

Skin Absorption of Toxic Chemicals in Water

Drinking water is not the only way toxic chemicals from water can enter the body.

Skin absorption (e.g. through bathing) is another viable route.

In fact, more chemicals may be absorbed during bathing than drinking the same water.

CONCERNS

Parents may not be aware that water in their home can have different contaminants than water tested at the municipal site.

Parents may be buying bottled water that is, in fact, not pure water at all.

Parents may think they are eliminating the risks associated with contaminated water by giving their families filtered drinking water.

Parents may not realize that their family can also absorb toxic chemicals as they bathe daily.

Reducing Water Contaminants

SOLUTIONS

Home Water Analysis

The water in your home can be tested by purchasing a kit.

Water samples are then sent to an independent company.

The company will then provide you an unbiased, specific analysis of your water (versus what it may be at the municipal plant).

A reputable company which tests water is:

Watercheck National Testing Laboratories, Inc.

6151 Willson Mills Road

Cleveland, Ohio 44133

Water Systems

The type of preferred system depends largely on the quality of water (tested at the tap).

Systems and filters may be installed at any individual faucet or shower.

Systems can also be purchased for an entire home where the water from all faucets and showers is filtered.

Companies

Reputable companies offering such systems are:

E.L. Foust
Box 105
Elmhust, IL 60126
1-800-225-9549

Environmental Purification Systems
P.O. Box 191
Concord, CA 94522
(800) 829-2129

When No filtered Water is Available

Until a water system can be installed, boiling water can help reduce some water contamination.

Water boiled in a glass pot for 10 minutes is effective for removing chlorine and chlorine by-products and killing bacteria.

Medicine and Your Child

Many people do not realize that drugs and medicine represent a major form of chemical and toxic ingestion for children. We tend to think of medicines as benign and helpful, which of course, in the right circumstances, they certainly are. However, it is important to realize just how powerful these chemicals in the form of drugs can be, so that the child can be protected from excessive amounts through careful consideration.

It is a useful exercise to actually read some of the warning labels and warning inserts provided by even the most common over the counter drugs, such as acetominophen (a common pain reliever) or some of the cough syrups, etc.

Of course, when a child is running a high fever or is otherwise very sick, our first impulse is to obtain help from doctors and their medicines. In order to not put the child at any kind of risk, many people are certainly cautious in this regard and this is understood and appreciated.

So is there anything that can be done to minimize the impact of these chemicals on the children, without increasing the fear of failing to deal with the illness effectively according to the best light we have?

The answer to this is a qualified "yes". It involves exercising understanding and insight into the disease process and trying to avoid the use of drugs in those cases where the risk is low and the alternatives are relatively effective. By reducing reliance on chemical drugs in terms of the day to day problems, we reserve their use for those cases where there are no really acceptable and effective alternatives readily available.

WHAT OPTIONS ARE AVAILABLE?

Herbs and Herbal Remedies: herbs have been in use for thousands of years around the world as natural healing substances. They are considered to be concentrated nutritional or energetic foods with a tremendous, yet gentle, power of healing. There are a number of books available about herbal lore and herbs are widely available in health food stores around the country or by mail order. Some, such as chamomile, can be found as herbal teas in almost any supermarket.

Homeopathy

During the late 1800's and early 1900's homeopathy enjoyed a wide following in this country. It is recognized as a valid medical science and has its own U.S. pharmacopeia for homeopathic remedies. Homeopathy is an "energetic" healing science which believes that the more a substance is diluted the stronger it can act on the subtle energetics of the body such that the response of the body is more intense and effective. The basic principle is that a substance is used that would in ordinary course produce the symptoms in evidence. The "potentized" form of this substance (that is, more diluted), evokes a response from the body and the patient essentially "heals himself" from this response. Homeopathy is known as a gentle healing science.

Flower Remedies

Traditional English Flower Remedies developed in the tradition of Dr. Edward Bach are well-known homeopathic remedies useful particularly in cases of emotional distress of various sorts. The uses of the Rescue or Emergency Remedy is legendary for helping deal with trauma or accident or any kind of disturbed atmosphere which is upsetting to the child.

Naturopathy

Also known as "nature cure", this healing practice essentially believes that an intelligent relationship of the mind and body to the issue of health can maintain and restore health without the use of a lot of drugs. This practice will rely on exercise, diet, fresh air and positive attitude to enhance the natural health. There is a lot of emphasis on understanding the needs of the body and providing appropriate healthy nutrition and avoiding the poisons and toxins of the society.

Infant Massage

There are numerous proponents of the view that the stimulation and attention provided by systematic and regular infant massage will help the child respond more effectively to its environment in a healthy manner.

SOURCES

Books and Information: Health Food Stores or Alternative Bookstores should have extensive information about herbs, homeopathy, alternative health practices, and massage techniques, as well as the issue of the toxicity of drugs and medicines.

Some fine books in the field include:

Guide to Homeopathy

Homeopathy and Your Child

Planetary Herbology

Herbal Formulas that Work

Bach Flower Therapy

Bach Flower Remedies to the Rescue

PRODUCTS

Hyland's/Standard Homeopathic features a number of homeopathic products for children and a "First Aid Kit" for children.

A wide assortment of Herbs and Herbal Products, as well as homeopathic products and Books are available from:

Wholesale: Lotus Light Distributing

P O Box 1008 NTB, Silver Lake, WI 53170

414/889-8501

Retail: Lotus Fulfilment Service
33719 116th Street, Dept. NTB
Twin Lakes, WI 53181

Rescue Remedy is available at many health food stores or you can write to:

Swanstar
Box 2596
Vista, CA 92085

BOOKS

(The following resource is able to mail order a large selection of books in the field if you are having trouble finding some of these texts locally)

Swanstar
Box 2596
Vista, CA 92085

Chemical Glossary

TEN CHEMICALS TO WHICH WE ARE COMMONLY EXPOSED

BENZENE

Found In: water near gasoline refineries, paint solvent, glues, cleaning fluids, gasoline

> *Health Concerns: Known to cause cancer and damage to human blood cells. Causes chromosome damage and birth defects in rats.*

BHA (Butylated Hydroxanisole) AND
BHT (Butylated Hydroxytoluene)

Found In: food and personal care products

> *Health Concerns: BHT causes cancer in animals and has shown to promote tumors in mice. Suspected of causing cancer in humans. Accumulates in human fat. BHA affects liver and kidney function. Some experts believe BHA and BHT cause hyperactivity and behavioral disturbances in some children.*

CHLORINE

Found In: water, laundry bleaches, swimming pools

> *Health Concerns: Combines with organic matter in water to produce cancer-causing compounds. Symptoms can include: red eyes, skin rashes, pain and inflammation of the mouth, and severe respiratory-tract irritation.*

DIOXIN

Found in: paper products, pesticide formulas, disposable diapers

> *Health Concerns: Strongly indicated in causing birth defects and liver damage.*

ETHANOL (also known as Ethyl Alcohol)

Found In: plastics, office fluids, cleaning products

> *Health Concerns: Can cause cerebral symptoms and central nervous system depression.*

FORMALDEHYDE

Found In: synthetic carpet, clothing, paint, nail polish, mouthwash, toothpaste, air fresheners, facial tissue, shampoo, adhesives, cosmetics, building materials, paper, plastic - over 85 common household items

> *Health Concerns: Known to cause cancer in animals. Recommended to be viewed as a potential human carcinogen. Symptoms from inhalation of vapors include: swelling of the throat, respiratory problems, headaches, disorientation, depression, and watery eyes.*

FRAGRANCES (can indicate up to 4.000 fragrances)

Found In: diapers, shampoos, toilet paper, detergents, perfumes, personal care products

> *Health Concerns: Symptoms include: headaches, dizziness, rashes, hyperactivity, irritability, and depression.*

NAPHTHALENE

Found In: laundry detergents

> *Health Concerns:: Suspected of causing cancer in humans. Symptoms include: skin irritation, headache, confusion.*

POLYCHLORINATED BIPHENYLS (PCBS)

Found In: electrical equipment

> *Health Concerns:: Accumulates in body tissue, specifically mother's milk. Has been linked to birth defects, liver problems, and chronic fatigue.*

VINYL CHLORIDE

Found in: toys, furniture, cars, foods wrapped in heat-sealed plastic

> *Health Concerns:: Causes cancer, birth defects, and genetic defects. Symptoms can include chronic bronchitis, mucous-membrane dryness, allergic skin reactions.*

BIBLIOGRAPHY

Begley, Sharon and Mary Hayer. "A Guide to Grocery." *Newsweek*. March 27,1989.

Bond, Anne Berthold. *Clean and Green: The Complete Guide to Nontoxicand Environmentally Safe Housekeeping.* Woodstock, NY: Ceres Publishing, 1990.

"Chemlawn Yields in New York Suit." *Pesticides and You.* Vo. 10, No. 3, August, 1990.

"Contaminated Mother's Milk." *The Human Ecologist.* No. 35, 1987.

Crook, William, M.D. *The Yeast Connection.* New York: Random House, 1986.

Dadd, Debra. *Nontoxic, Natural, and Earthwise.* Los Angeles, CA: Jeremy P. Tarcher, Inc., 1990.

"The Dioxin Connection." *Mothering.* No. 53, Fall 1989.

Goodman, Robert. *A Quick Guide to Food Additives.* San Diego, CA: Silvercat Publications, 1989.

Green, Nancy Sokol. *Poisioning Our Children: Surviving in a Toxic World.* Chicago: The Noble Press, Inc., 1991.

Heifetz, Dr. Ruth and Sharon Taylor. "Mother's Milk or Mother's Poison?" *Journal of Pesticide Reform.* Vol. 9, No. 3, Fall 1989.

Hunter, Beatrice Trum. "Diet and Health for Children." *The Human Ecologist.* Fall, 1990.

The Inside Story: A Guide to Indoor Air Quality. Washington, D.C.; United States Environmental Protection Agency, United States Consumer Product Safety Commission, 1988.

Kosta, Louise. "The Sad Legacy of Lead." *The Human Ecologist.* Winter, 1990.

Lappe, Frances Moore. *Diet for a Small Planet.* New York: Ballantine Books, 1982.

Mead, Mark. "Chlorination: Friend or Foe?" *East West.* Dec., 1989.

Mott. Lawrie and Karen Snyder. *Pesticide Alert.* San Francisco: Sierra Club, 1987.

Obrien, Mary. "But What About the Other Half?: The Fascinating Tale of the (Non) Inerts." *Journal of Pesticide Reform*. Summer, 1986.

Oski, Frank., M.D. *Don't Drink Your Milk*. Syracuse, NY: Mollica Press, 1983.

Robbins, John. *Diet for a New America*. Walpole, NH: Stillpoint Publishing, 1987.

Rogers, Sherry, M.D. *Tired or Toxic?* Syracuse, NY: Prestige Publishing, 1990.

Sellin, Mary. "The Mythology of Pesticide Safety." *NCAP News*. Spring/Summer, 1983.

"Skin Absorption: An Important Route of Exposure." *Toxiformer*. San Diego, CA: Environmental Health Coalition. May/June, 1989.

Steinman, David. "How I Came Clean." *California*. June, 1990.

Tattersall, Ann. "Is EPA Registration a Guarantee of Pesticide Safety?" *Jounal of Pesticide Reform*. Spring, 1986.

Weir, David. and Mark. Shapiro. *Circle of Poison*. San Francisco: Institute for Food and Development Policy, 1981.

Additional copies of **The Nontoxic Baby** can be ordered from:

Natural Choices, Box 2596, Vista, CA 92085 • 619/945-1050

Purchase price $9.95

Add $2.00 for tax and shipping

NATURAL CHOICES

P. O. Box 2596

Vista, CA 92085

619/945-1050

Natural Choices was created to present references, solutions, alternatives and products which enable families to easily substitute toxic lifestyles for nontoxic living.

We hope that as more people recognize the problems associated with a polluted planet, they will also make the connection that humans are part of that same environment. With that connection. we are confident more people will discover that nontoxic living ensures a healthy planet, and that a nontoxic planet ensures a healthy population.

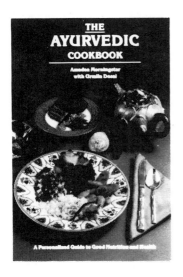

THE
AYURVEDIC
COOKBOOK

by Amadea Morningstar
with Urmila Desai

Introduction by Dr. David Frawley

$18.95 (postpaid); 340 pp.; 6 x 9,
paper; ISBN: 0-914955-06-3

The Ayurvedic Cookbook gives a fresh new
perspective on this ancient art of self-
healing. Over 250 taste-tested recipes
specifically designed to balance each
constitution, with an emphasis on simplicity, ease and sound nutrition. Designed for
the Western diner, recipes range from exotic Indian meals to old American favorites.
Amadea Morningstar, M.A., a Western trained nutritionist, and Urmila Desai, a superb
Indian cook, are both well-versed in a variety of healing traditions. *The Ayurvedic
Cookbook* includes an in-depth discussion of Ayurvedic nutrition, *tridoshic* perspectives
and ways to make dietary changes that last.

"This is not just another recipe book, but a unique health manual that, if applied
with proper understanding, can lead to a whole new dimension in the enhancement of
health and the joy of eating."

Yogi Amrit Desai
Founder, Kripalu Center, Spiritual Director

"This book, inspired by the Ayurvedic science of nutrition, can help readers learn
how to use food to enhance the quality of their lives."

Dr. Robert Svoboda, Ayurvedic physician
Author, *Prakruti, Your Ayurvedic Constitution*

"This book reveals simple recipes based upon Ayurvedic principles which can serve
a guide for an individual in his daily cooking."

Dr. Vasant Lad, Ayurvedic physician
Author, *Ayurveda, The Science of Self-Healing*
Co-author, *The Yoga of Herbs* (with Dr. David Frawley)

To order your copy, send $18.95 (postpaid) to:

Lotus Press
P.O. Box 325-NTB
Twin Lakes, WI 53181
Request our complete book & sidelines catalog.
Wholesale inquiries welcome.

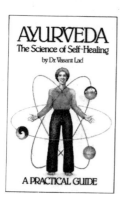

AYURVEDA
The Science of Self-Healing
A PRACTICAL GUIDE
by Dr. Vasant Lad,
Ayurvedic Physician

For the first time a book is available which clearly explains the principles and practical applications of Ayurveda, the oldest healing system in the world.

The text contains 176 well-illustrated pages which thoroughly explain the following:

History & Philosophy	First Aid
Basic Principles	Food Antidotes
Diagnostic Techniques	Medicinal Usage of
Treatment	Kitchen Herbs & Spices
Diet	And Much More

More than 50 concise charts, diagrams and tables are included, as well as a glossary and index in order to further clarify the text.

Dr. Vasant Lad, a native of India, has been a practitioner and professor of Ayurvedic Medicine for more than 20 years. He conducts the only full-time program of study on Ayurveda in the United States as Program Director of The Ayurvedic Institute in Albuquerque, New Mexico. In addition, Dr. Lad has lectured extensively throughout the U.S., and has written numerous published articles on Ayurveda.